Yoga For Men

*Beginner's Step by Step Guide to
a Stronger Body & Sharper Mind*

TABLE OF CONTENTS

INTRODUCTION

I want to thank you for reading my book, '*Yoga for Men: Beginner's Step by Step Guide to a Stronger Body & Sharper Mind*' and hope you find the book informative and interesting.

This book contains a step-by-guide on yoga for men. Particularly, here, you can learn the *basics of yoga, breathing techniques, yoga poses,* and *yoga sequences* – all for men! Other than that, you can even learn how to create and implement your own yoga routine.

If this is your first take at yoga, don't worry; this book will teach you the essentials from a beginner's perspective. By the end of the five chapters, chances are, you can't wait for your new yoga routine to commence. Granted you stick to the instructions, you'll easily learn the ropes.

Thanks again for reading my book, I hope you enjoy it!

CHAPTER 1

YOGA FOR MEN:
AN INTRODUCTION

A common reason that the manliest of men are into yoga? It comes with a roster of superb benefits; it's a plus for physical and mental wellness. Not only does it grant them a fit body, it also rewards them with a calm and relaxed mind. Even those who used to think that the poses and sequences are for girls and are overrated, as well as those who were against the practice before… They are now proud yogis.

Understand Yoga & That It is for Men, too

Since men's workouts are often associated with masculine activities such as lifting heavy weights and performing a grand number of push-ups, the idea of yoga for men is quite questionable. While some choose not to engage in it with it appearing as an unsatisfying exercise regimen, other men insist on adopting a yoga routine for its overall health benefits.

According to a 2013 research about yoga being an exercise for both genders, yoga is a plus as much for men as it is for women. From an outsider's perspective, its physical satisfaction may not be obvious; it seems as if all a yogi does is chill and do some stretching. However, for the *man* yogi, he can gradually experience the positive impacts of yoga for his physical and mental wellbeing.

There are certain misconceptions that exist about yoga, especially in the minds of men. Do you feel that yoga is a girly form of exercise? Well, don't just visualize women in spandex doing stretches. That's not what yoga is about. It is a well-balanced form of exercise that helps to create harmony between your body and mind. Various male celebrities swear by yoga like Russell Brand, Colin Farrell, Matthew

McConaughey, Richard Gere and Robert Downey Jr. Well, if Iron Man likes yoga, so can you! Yoga does have spiritual undertones, but it is not a religion. So, don't be under any misconceptions about that! Another popular misconception is that men think they cannot perform all the twisty bends. Let me stop you right there. You never know how flexible your body is until you try. Don't worry about what others think. Practice yoga because it is good for you.

Well, if you have any of these misconceptions, then you will undoubtedly change your mind after you read about the different benefits yoga offers.

Body + Mind & Other Perks

For a strong body, men shouldn't set aside the advantages of yoga. By adhering to a regular yoga routine, he will be privileged to a boost in his overall physical function. If he is troubled with certain illnesses such as *arthritis, kidney problems, respiratory ailments, prostate cancer, cardiovascular complications,* and other physiological diseases, practicing yoga may help. Compared to rigorous gym sessions, its approach can seem a bit dull and *unconventional* for most of the guys, but nonetheless, it is linked to numerous health perks for the physical wellbeing.

Since it works with the nervous system (particularly, the parasympathetic and sympathetic nervous system), yoga promotes the wellness of the mind. It causes a dramatic improvement in one's mood and soothes his spirit. For those dealing with *social phobia, anxiety, depression,* and *mood swings,* performing yoga poses and sequences can help.

Additionally, yoga increases *libido.* Since many of the poses regulate blood flow and improve blood circulation near the groin area, men get to perform well in bed. Other than that, with the exercises boosting their concentration and energy levels, they become more responsive sexual partners. It's no surprise that most of them who are into yoga have incredible sex lives.

There are so many benefits that yoga offers. Some benefits are quite evident, and the rest are subtle. When you put them all together, it improves your overall wellbeing.

Better flexibility

If you move and stretch your muscles, your flexibility will improve. You can start to feel a better range of motions even in the tight areas. After a while, you can experience flexibility in your hamstrings, back, shoulders and hips as well. With age, the flexibility of your muscles decreases, especially if you sit for a long time and it leads to pain as well as immobility. With the help of yoga, you can successfully reverse this process.

Develops strength

The yoga poses might seem deceptively simple. I mean, how difficult can it be to stretch your body? Well, don't be under any false impressions that yoga is just about stretching your body. Most of the yoga poses make use of your body weight in different ways. When you perform the tree pose where you have to support your body weight on one leg or when you have to support your body weight with just your arms in the downward facing dog, it takes time, practice and considerable strength to hold these poses. You will be able to develop your muscle strength without even realizing that you are in fact doing so.

Better muscle tone and definition

Yoga doesn't help you to bulk up. However, it does help to build lean muscle and tone your body. Your muscle tone improves with yoga. It helps to shape all the lean and long muscles in your body like your legs, arms, back, and abdomen. When you decide to lift weights to bulk up at the gym, you tend to lose flexibility. However, with yoga, you can develop six pack abs and maintain your muscle tone! If you want a well-defined body, then yoga is the best form of exercise.

Balance

Yoga requires balance. A significant benefit is the improvement of balance if you do yoga regularly. Not just that, it helps you to develop your core strength as well.

Joint health

Yoga requires you to perform movements that are of low intensity. It means that you can use your joints without doing them any damage. It strengthens the muscles around your joints and lessens the load on these muscles. If you have arthritis, then you indeed cannot perform any HIIT exercises. However, you can do yoga without any worry. It improves your mobility and strengthens your joints.

No lower back pains

We all lead hectic lifestyles these days. Most of us tend to spend a lot of time hunched in front of our laptops. When you do this, you put a lot of pressure on your lower back. Therefore, it is no wonder that lower back problems are quite common. Even when you spend a lot of time driving, you will notice a sort of tightness all over your body. Your posture can lead to spinal compression and yoga counteracts all this. Certain yoga poses can reduce your lower back pain like the cobra pose.

Improved breathing

We tend to take shallow breaths usually. In fact, most of us don't concentrate on how we breathe. Yoga has plenty of breathing exercises that will force you to focus on how you breathe. For instance, pranayama is all about conscious breathing. When you breathe properly, your body has an uninterrupted and a steady flow of oxygen. A better supply of oxygen will make you more active. Not just that it helps to clear up your nasal passages and even calm your nervous system. You will learn about the different benefits of breathing exercises in the coming chapters.

Mental calmness

The practice of yoga asanas is mostly physical. When you start to concentrate on what your body does, it tends to make your mind calm. Meditation techniques are a significant part of yoga as well. When you focus on the way you breathe, you won't obsess on your thoughts. All this can make you calm. When your mind is calm, you can reorganize your thoughts. You can also disengage from thinking anything negative. You cannot practice yoga when you are distracted. Intense concentration is a precondition to practicing yoga.

Reduces stress

Any form of physical activity is helpful to relieve stress, even more so when you practice yoga. You have to concentrate, and therefore all your daily problems, big and small, seemingly melt away when you do yoga. While on the yoga mat, you won't be able to think about all the unnecessary troubles that weigh you down. It provides you with a clean break from all the stress you experience daily. Yoga places great emphasis on the present moment, and you won't have the time to think about past or future events. After a session of yoga, you will feel less stressed.

Self-confidence

Yoga improves the connection between your body, mind, and soul. It makes you aware of your body. Yoga helps you to learn to make subtle movements that help in better alignment of your body and mind. It helps you to form a bond with your physical and mental being. You also learn to accept your body without any judgments. When you can fully accept your body, you will feel more comfortable in your skin. All this helps to boost your self-confidence.

Common Yoga Terms Defined

Before they get into yoga, men should be familiar with certain terminologies; they should be familiar with *Sanskrit* words that will often be used throughout yoga sessions. Regardless if they choose to perform yoga on their own or if they prefer to sign up for a pro-yoga teacher's classes, they won't easily scratch their heads upon encounter with common yoga terms.

The list of common Sanskrit words:

- Asana – a term used to describe a yoga pose
- Mudra – it means the movement or space between asanas
- Namaste - a salutation used by most yoga instructors
- Om – a mantra recited during yoga practices
- Prana - a term used to describe energy or a life force
- Pranayama – a term used to describe breathing techniques

5 Yogic Techniques

Many men who are yoga beginners think that all the asanas are one and the same. Since they all look like they belong in a category of stretching methods, they are classified exactly as that: *stretching methods*. However, the reason why there are different asanas is there are different yogic techniques, too. For the achievement of total wellness, each one is focused on giving importance to one's prana.

Different yogic techniques:

1. Bikram yogic technique – performed in a heated room
2. Hatha yoga – based on basic poses; often thought as a general meditation technique; focused on relaxation
3. Iyengar yoga – can be physically and mentally demanding; promotes speed and accuracy; focused on the proper *pranayamas*
4. Kripalu – divided into three parts; promotes awareness of individual limits; quite experimental
5. Restorative yogic technique – often thought as any yogic technique that is neither physically nor mentally demanding; focused on relaxation and psychic cleansing

Beginner Mistakes

A common beginner misconception about yoga is that it is easy; some men, especially those who have only seen it done by TV personalities, think it's simply about extending the arms and legs. Alongside, there are people who assume that any time and any way preferred it could be accomplished. According to the more serious yogis, the effective practice of yoga should be done with regard to certain regulations. Adopting the "correct" way of performing yoga sequences can take time.

On a related note, yes yoga is *easy*. However, it's not usually easy at the beginning. You have to stay committed to learning about the proper way to perform different *pranayamas* and *asanas*; granted, you'll eventually get the hang of the practice.

Important reminders:

- Always observe the alignment of your body parts
- Avoid food and drinks before practicing yoga
- Begin with basic and easy asanas; look at the picture of a pose and use it as a basis whether or not it is doable
- Consult a doctor if you're experiencing discomfort or certain health-related concerns (e.g. high blood pressure, bone fractures, injuries)
- In case you experience pain, do not ignore it - especially if you don't think it's reasonable to suffer pain in a particular body part

Tools, Setting & Attire

If you want to practice the different asanas with the items you currently own, you have the freedom. There's no need to shop for a set of tools and spend more than $100 bucks; your belongings at home will do. Remember, yoga is rather flexible; you can do it on your own or with a group; just keep a few reminders noted.

Important reminders:

- Be ready with a *yoga belt, yoga block, yoga mat,* and *yoga towel*; this allows you to accomplish some poses accordingly.
- Go with absorbent and breathable clothing; this guarantees comfort during sessions.
- Go with tight or form-fitting shirts and shorts/pants; this allows you to evaluate your progress (i.e. whether the body is aligned properly).
- Practice yoga in a spacious environment; this allows freedom of movement.

CHAPTER 2

BREATHING EXERCISES

Before setting forth to practice yoga, men should learn about different yogic breathing techniques. Contrary to others' opinion, the practice is not all about adopting a particular pose and breathing as desired. This is where the need for patience is emphasized; yoga seems easy but if you get around to it, it can be nerve-racking.

Moreover, the practice of yoga *requires discipline*; to achieve overall wellness, you should turn to the rules of proper pranayama. And, as the more experienced practitioners' advice goes, learn to take it a step at a time; eventually, you will receive the health benefits of the practice.

About Pranayama

The breathing exercise or pranayama is a brilliant way to start your day. The best time to practice pranayama is early in the morning. It is even better if you can practice pranayama outdoors. Nothing else can make you feel as good as fresh air in the morning. If you want to do pranayama in the morning, then do so on an empty stomach. In this section, you will learn about the different benefits of pranayama.

Leads to detoxification

Did you know that your body tends to release about 70% of all the toxins through breathing? If you don't breathe efficiently, you stop your body from efficiently releasing all the pent-up toxins. It means that the pressure on all the other systems in the body will increase and it can cause illnesses as well. The natural waste of your body's metabolism is carbon dioxide. Your body releases carbon dioxide whenever you exhale.

Releases tension as well

How does your body feel when you are angry, tensed or scared? Does your body feel constricted? Does it feel like the muscles in your body are tensing up? Your muscles become tight, and your breathing becomes quite shallow. Your body doesn't get the necessary oxygen when your breathing is shallow. So, deep breathing helps to cleanse the system and relax your muscles. Thereby, it helps to release tension as well. Not just that, it helps to bring clarity to your emotions as well.

Relaxes mind and body

When your brain gets sufficient oxygen, it helps to reduce the anxiety levels. Pay attention to the way you breathe. Take in slow and deep breaths. When you inhale, concentrate on the action of inhalation and nothing else. Notice all those spots in your body that feel tight and wound up. Deep breathing helps to relax your body as well as the mind.

Massages your organs

Did you know that there is a connection between how you think, feel and your perspective towards life? For instance, how does your body react when it anticipates pain? Your body tenses up, and you hold your breath. If you practice deep breathing, you can reduce the pain that you experience. Don't let your body tense up. Your diaphragm moves during pranayama, and it helps to massage various internal organs like the stomach, liver, pancreas, small intestine, and heart as well. It indirectly helps to improve the circulation of blood to these organs. Several breathing exercises can help you to tone the abdominal muscles as well.

It helps to increase the muscle in the body and strengthens the immune system. Hemoglobin is a pigment in blood that absorbs oxygen and transports it to all the cells in the body. When there is an increase in the supply of oxygen, it enriches your body. Breathing exercises help to improve your overall mood.

Getting ready for pranayama

East or north is the best direction to do pranayama. So, pick a spot that faces north or east. Place your yoga mat on the floor and sit cross-legged. Make sure that you stretch your spine, and your head, neck, and chest are correctly aligned. You shouldn't perform pranayama after you eat, bathe, or engage in any sexual activity. There should be a gap of at least an hour. Pranayama is quite easy to perform. However, certain people shouldn't perform it. Pregnant women or those on their menstrual cycle should abstain from it. If you have any heart condition or recently had a cardiac arrest, then you shouldn't perform pranayama. All those with low blood pressure shouldn't perform it without the supervision of a teacher or a doctor. If you are ill or have fever, bronchitis, and pneumonia, abstain from pranayama until you get better. Anyone who is undergoing chemo or radiation therapy is exempt from the list as well. It isn't recommended for anyone who has any psychological conditions either. If you have any pre-existing medical conditions, it is better than you get a certificate of clearance from your doctor or physician if you want to do pranayama.

Before you move onto advanced pranayama techniques like Bhasktrika, you should start with more straightforward exercises like Nadi shodhona. Nadi shodhona helps to purify the nervous system. The best method to start with is the alternate nostril breathing.

Alternate nostril breathing

The Sanskrit name of alternate nostril breathing technique is anuloma viloma. As the name suggests, this pranayama exercise requires you to breathe through the alternate nostrils of your nose. You will primarily be breathing only through one nostril at a time. It is a part of Nadi shodhona or the purification of the nervous system. To perform this exercise, find a comfortable spot for yourself. You can either sit on the floor or a chair with your feet firmly placed on the floor. Start to take deep breaths with your left nostril. Do this ten times and then shift to the other nostril. It doesn't take more than 5 minutes to perform this calming exercise.

When you perform anuloma villoma, keep one of your nostrils closed at all times. You have to make use of your right hand's thumb, ringer finger, and little finger to close your nostril. To close your right nostril, use your thumb. To close your left nostril, use your ring and little fingers. Keep your mouth shut and don't inhale or exhale through your mouth. Don't make any sounds while you inhale or exhale.

Practice

There are two rounds to practice this technique. In the first round, start by focusing on your breath for a minute. Observe how air flows from both your nostrils. Raise your right hand and form the pranayama mudra.

Lift your right hand such that your thumb, little finger, and ring finger are pointing outwards. The other two fingers should be bent inwards. Keep your thumb gently on the right nostril and close it and inhale from the left nostril. Once you inhale, you have to close your left nostril with the ring and little finger. Only after you close your left nostril, can you exhale through the right one. After you exhale from your right nostril, inhale from the same one. To exhale, you have to close the right nostril and let go of your breath through the left one. To simplify it all, in the first round, you have to perform the following four steps.

- Inhale through the left nostril
- Exhale from the right nostril
- Inhale from the right nostril, and
- Then exhale from the left nostril.

After ten rounds, place your hand on your knee and concentrate on your breathing for a minute. For round two, you have to position your left hand in the pranayama mudra. Repeat the steps mentioned above, but with the other nostril.

So, you will start to inhale with your right nostril, exhale through the left one, then inhale through the same nostril, and finally exhale through the right nostril. After you perform ten rounds, place your hand on your knee and focus on your breathing for a minute. It is as simple as that.

There are various benefits of this exercise. You will feel at peace and relaxed. It is believed that this form of pranayama helps to clear 72000 channels of nadis in the human body. If you want to purify your respiratory system, then this is the best breathing exercise. It helps to reduce stress and anxiety and offers all the other benefits that were discussed earlier.

Practice *Pranayamas* or Different Yogic Breathing Techniques

There are different pranayamas or yogic breathing techniques since yogis have varying preferences. Nonetheless, the goal of breathing accordingly should remain; the focus must be on proper inhalation and exhalation, rather than which method seems better. Granted that the air in the surroundings is not polluted, try practicing the set of breathing techniques daily.

The techniques:

1. Abdominal Breathing

    Benefits:
    calms mind; reduces stress; strengthens abdominal muscles

    Level:
    easy

    Directions:
    1. Place one hand on chest; place the other hand on belly.
    2. Inhale deeply through the nostrils; make sure that the diaphragm is inflated.
    3. Breathe slowly and deeply for about 15 minutes.

2. Progressive Relaxation

    Benefits:
    relaxes muscles all over the body

    Level:
    easy

    Directions:
    1. Close eyes and focus on muscle groups.
    2. For about 5 seconds, focus on the muscles in the feet; take slow and deep breaths through your nose.
    3. Do the same for the other muscles in the knees, lower and upper thighs, chest, hands, arms, neck, and face.

3. Equal Breathing

    Benefits:
    calms mind; finds body balance; relaxes muscles all over the body

Level:

easy

Directions:
1. Close eyes.
2. Inhale deeply through your nose for about 5 seconds.
3. Exhale deeply through your nose for about 5 seconds.
4. Perform technique for about 10 minutes.

4. Breathe & Squeeze

Benefits:

calms mind; reduces stress; strengthens arms, back, and pelvic floor

Level:

easy

Directions:
1. Stand straight.
2. Inhale deeply through your nose for about 5 seconds; make sure that the lower abdomen is contracting.
3. Exhale deeply through your nose for about 5 seconds; make sure that the pelvic muscles are "squeezing".
4. Perform technique for about 10 minutes.

5. Kalapabhati

Benefits:

boosts energy; calms mind; strengthens abdominal muscles

Level:

easy

Directions:
1. Stand straight.
2. Inhale and exhale deeply through your nose for about 3 minutes.
3. Inhale and exhale more deeply through your nose for about 3 minutes.
4. Continue raising the breathing intensity (as much as possible) every 3 minutes.
5. Perform technique for about 15 minutes.

6. Guided Visualization

Benefits:

calms mind; relaxes muscles all over the body

Level:

easy

Directions:
1. Focus on a goal; picture the goal's achievement.
2. Inhale and exhale deeply through your nose.
3. Perform technique for about 5 minutes.

7. Nadi Shodhona

Benefits:

calms mind; finds body balance

Level:

beginner

Directions:
1. Place left hand over left nostril.
2. Inhale deeply through right nostril for about 5 seconds.
3. Exhale.
4. Do the same for the opposite side; place right hand over right nostril, inhale deeply through left nostril for about 5 seconds, and exhale.
5. Perform technique 10 times for each nostril.

8. Alligator Breathing

Benefits:

calms mind; reduces upper body's stress; strengthens diaphragms

Level:

intermediate

Directions:
1. Lie on the belly.
2. Inhale deeply through your nose as torso is raised above the floor.
3. Once torso is raised, exhale deeply through your nose.
4. Perform technique 10 times.

9. Drop and Arch

   Benefits:
   calms mind; improves circulation; increases resistance level

   Level:
   intermediate

   Directions:
   1. Go into kneeling position; make sure that back is flat.
   2. Inhale and exhale deeply through your nose.
   3. Perform technique for about 5 minutes.

10. Intercostals Breathing

    Benefits:
    calms mind; reduces stress; relaxes muscles all over the body

    Level:
    intermediate

    Directions:
    1. Drape left hand over your head.
    2. Stretch right hand towards the ceiling.
    3. Inhale and exhale deeply through your nose.
    4. Perform technique for about 15 minutes.

Note: Always keep your mouth closed while you perform any of these techniques; unless it is explicitly mentioned to do otherwise.

CHAPTER 3

40 YOGA POSES FOR MEN

According to yoga experts, one of the advantages of attending yoga practice sessions and being greeted *Namaste* regularly is that it is revitalizing; there is nary a doubt that men can benefit from yoga, and with carefully selected poses, the benefits can be maximized. Given the fact that men's body structure differs from women's, they should go for poses that are designed for their gender. Alongside, the majority of men need to work out *specific muscles* (e.g. hamstrings and hips); otherwise, they can be susceptible to weaknesses of sorts in certain areas. Thus, they could use a heads-up. In this chapter, the suggested list of men's yoga poses will be covered.

Be Familiar with Various Yoga Poses

While some of them don't find anything wrong with simple poses, many men prefer the more complicated poses since they like to challenge themselves. With some of them belonging to the group that can exhibit *short attention spans* to plain workouts (i.e. workouts that won't make them produce buckets of sweat). Nonetheless, becoming familiar with various yoga poses is a great beginners' approach. You may practice one pose per day or a series of poses; it's up to you.

Various yoga poses for men:

Level I Yoga Poses

1. Head to Knee Bend (or *Janu Sirsasana*)

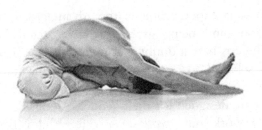

Benefits:

calms mind; eases knee and ankle injuries; improves flexibility; reduces stress

Equipment:

yoga mat

Level:

easy

Directions:

I. On your yoga mat, sit straight with your legs in front of you.

II. Inhale through your nose.

III. Bend or bring your right knee inward.

IV. Exhale through your nose.

V. Bend forward. Make sure that your head is somewhere near your knee. Maybe you cannot do so initially, after a little practice you will be able to.

VI. Stay in position for about 5 seconds.

2. Hands to Heart (or *Anjali Mudra*)

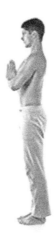

Benefits:
    calms mind; corrects posture; improves balance, focus, and
    memory; reduces stress

Equipment:
    yoga mat

Level:
    easy

Directions:
    I. Stand straight with feet together.
    II. Gently bring hands together toward your heart. Make it as
    if you are praying.
    III. Inhale and exhale deeply through your nose.

3. Wind-Relieving Pose (or *Pavanamuktasana*)

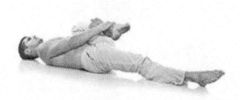

Benefits:
    promotes body detoxification; regulates digestive processes; relaxes spine; strengthens abdominal muscles

Equipment:
    yoga mat

Level:
    easy

Directions:
    I. On your yoga mat, lie on your back. Extend your legs and arms.
    II. Inhale through your nose.
    III. Draw one of your knees to your chest. Use your hands for support.
    IV. Exhale through your nose.
    V. Stay in position for about 10 seconds.

4. Hero Pose (or *Virasana*)

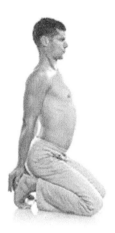

Benefits:
  calms mind; corrects posture; eases knee and ankle injuries; strengthens upper thighs

Equipment:
  yoga mat

Level:
  intermediate

Directions:
  I. Go into kneeling position.
  II. Keep your back straight and let your buttocks rest on your soles.
  III. Place your hands behind your back and touch the back of your feet.
  IV. Inhale and exhale deeply through your nose. Don't breathe in through your mouth, unless it is specifically mentioned.

5. Standing Forward Bend (or *Uttansana*)

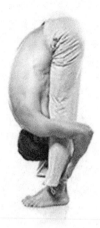

Benefits:

    calms mind; improves the flexibility of thighs and arms; reduces stress; strengthens hip and back muscles; stretches hamstrings

Equipment:

    yoga mat; yoga belt

Level:

    easy

Directions:

    I. On your yoga mat, stand straight.
    II. Gently bend down and reach for your toes. You may use yoga belt for better support.
    III. Secure the bend by holding the back of your ankles.
    IV. Remain in position; inhale and exhale deeply.

6. Pose of Infinity (or *Ananthasana*)

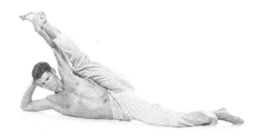

Benefits:

boosts immunity; improves flexibility of the hamstrings; promotes body detoxification; relaxes liver and spleen

Equipment:

yoga mat

Level:

easy

Directions:

I. Lie on your right side. Rest your head on your hand.
II. Gently raise your leg overhead. Hold onto the back of the hamstring.
III. Lift your kneecaps.
IV. Stay in position for about 15 seconds.

7. Knee to Chest Pose (or *Pavanamuktasana*)

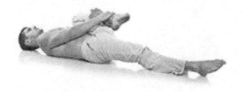

Benefits:
calms mind; eases knee and ankle injuries; improves balance; reduces stress
Equipment:
  yoga mat

Level:
  easy

Directions:
  I. On your yoga mat, lie on your back.
  II. Gently draw your left knee towards your chest as you inhale through your nose.
  III. Secure your position by placing your hand below your kneecap.
  IV. Exhale through your nose.
  V. Stay in position for about 10 seconds.

8.   Scale Pose (or *Tolasana*)

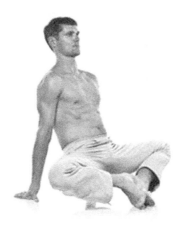

Benefits:
   eases ankle and knee injuries; improves the flexibility of back
   muscles; reduces stress; strengthens hips and thigh muscles

Equipment:
   yoga mat

Level:
   easy

Directions:
   I. Sit in a cross-legged position on your yoga mat.
   II. Place your palms on the floor. Make sure that they are
   beside your hips.
   III. Push your hands against the floor and exhale.
   IV. Contract your abdominal muscles.
   V. Slowly lift your buttocks and legs away from the floor.
   VI. Stay in position for about 15 seconds.
   VII. Slowly lower your buttocks and legs to the floor.
   VIII. Stay in position for about 5 seconds.

9. Bridge Pose (or *Setu Bandha Naukasana*)

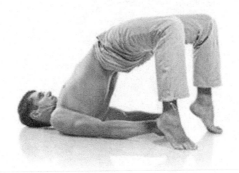

Benefits:
   boosts energy; calms mind; increases the flexibility of leg muscles

Equipment:
   yoga mat; yoga belt

Level:
   easy

Directions:
   I. On top of a yoga mat, lie down on back.
   II. Bend knees as feet are positioned flatly on the ground.
   III. Use yoga belt for support. Gently raise hips.
   IV. Position both hands underneath.
   V. Inhale and exhale deeply through your nose.

10. Bow Pose (or *Urdva Chakrasana*)

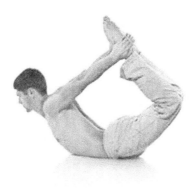

Benefits:
    improves blood circulation, focus, and memory; strengthens back, legs, and thighs

Equipment:
    yoga mat; yoga belt

Level:
    easy

Directions:
    I. On your yoga mat, lie down on your belly.
    II. Keep hands at the side of the chest.
    III. Inhale and exhale deeply through your nose.
    IV. You may use your yoga belt for better support. Slowly raise legs; reach legs with both hands.
    V. Inhale and exhale deeply through your nose.

11. Chair Pose (or *Utkatasana*)

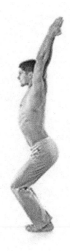

Benefits:
    calms mind; improves balance, focus, and memory; reduces stress

Equipment:
    yoga mat

Level:
    easy

Directions:
    I. On your yoga mat, stand straight with feet together.
    II. Raise both hands.
    III. Inhale through your nose while gently lowering your body. Lower your body as if you are sitting on a chair's edge.
    IV. Exhale through your nose.
    V. Stay in position for about 5 seconds.

12. Cat Pose (or *Marjaryasana*)

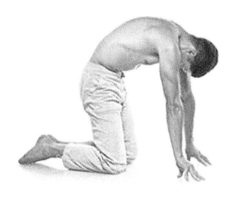

Benefits:

calms mind; eases ankle and knee injuries; improves focus; strengthens back muscles

Equipment:

yoga mat

Level:

easy

Directions:

I. On your yoga mat, kneel down and support yourself with your hands.

II. Face downward and arch your back while your feet, knees, and arms are on the ground.

III. Inhale and exhale deeply through your nose.

IV. Stay in position for about 10 seconds.

13. Prone Cobra (or Prone *Bhujangasana*)

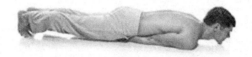

Benefits:
    calms mind; corrects posture; eases ankle and knee injuries;

Equipment:
    yoga mat

Level:
    easy

Directions:
    I. On your yoga mat, lie face down. Make sure your hands are resting on your body.
    II. Inhale and exhale deeply through your nose.
    III. Stay in position for about 10 seconds.

Level II Yoga Poses

14. Puppy Dog on Chair (or *Uttana Shishosana*)

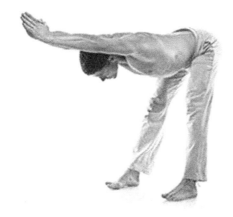

Benefits:
  calms mind; strengthens abdominal muscles

Equipment:
  yoga mat

Level:
  intermediate

Directions:
  I. Stand with feet slightly apart.
  II. Raise your hands over your head and press them together.
  III. Gently bend forward.
  IV. Inhale and exhale deeply through your nose.
  V. Stay in position for about 10 seconds.

15. Elevated Peacock Pose (or *Mayurasana Pincha*)

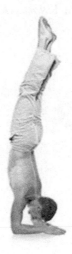

Benefits:
    calms mind; improves balance; reduces stress; relieves headache; strengthens upper arm and abdominal muscles

Equipment:
    yoga mat

Level:
    intermediate

Directions:
    I. On your yoga mat, go into kneeling position.
    II. Place your hands forward.
    III. Gently raise body upward and inhale deeply through your nose.
    IV. With your hands over your head, exhale deeply through your nose.

16. Warrior One Pose (or *Virabhadrasana*)

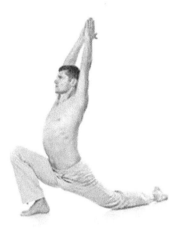

Benefits:
    finds body balance; improves the flexibility of legs and hips; strengthens butt, hips, and thighs

Equipment:
    yoga mat; yoga belt

Level:
    intermediate

Directions:
    I. On your yoga mat, stand straight.
    II. Place your left foot sideward.
    III. You may use your yoga belt for better support. Slowly raise both hands.
    IV. Inhale and exhale deeply through your nose.

17. Cobra Pose (or *Bhujangasana*)

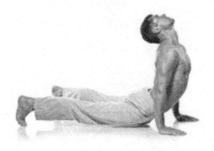

Benefits:
    calms mind; improves endurance; strengthens pelvic floor and feet

Equipment:
    yoga mat

Level:
    intermediate

Directions:
    I. On your yoga mat, lie down on your belly. Make sure that your legs spread.
    II. Gently rest forehead on the ground; make sure that shoulders are relaxed.
    III. Bend elbows and place forearms on the ground.
    IV. Inhale deeply through your nose while you raise your hips slowly.
    V. Exhale deeply through your nose while you lower your hips slowly.

18. Plow Pose (or *Halasana*)

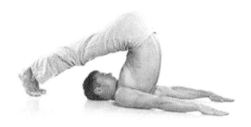

Benefits:
    finds body balance; improves the flexibility of legs; strengthens legs

Equipment:
    yoga mat

Level:
    intermediate

Directions:
    I. On your yoga mat, lie on back and slowly raise legs.
    II. Bring both legs backward; make sure that they are over your head.
    III. Place your hands at the back for support.
    IV. Inhale and exhale deeply through your nose.

19. Standing Hand to Big Toe Pose (or *Utthita Hasta Padangustanasana*)

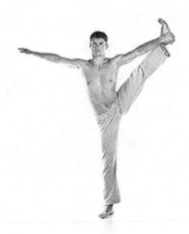

Benefits:
   boosts immunity; improves flexibility of the hamstrings; promotes body detoxification; relaxes liver and spleen

Equipment:
   yoga mat

Level:
   intermediate

Directions:
   I. On your yoga mat, stand straight.
   II. Extend your arms sideward.
   III. Gently raise your left leg and reach toward your left arm.
   IV. Inhale and exhale deeply through your nose.
   V. Stay in position for about 10 seconds.

20. Standing Quad Stretch

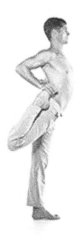

Benefits:

improves balance and flexibility; relaxes liver and spleen; strengthens arms, back, legs, and shoulders

Equipment:

yoga mat

Level:

intermediate

Directions:

I. On your yoga mat, stand straight.

II. Gently bend your right leg.

III. Secure the position with your right hand.

IV. Inhale and exhale deeply through your nose.

V. Stay in position for about 10 seconds.

21. Balancing Table (or *Dandayanma Bharmanasana*)

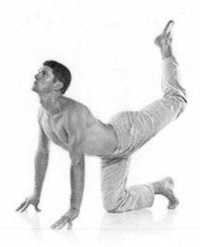

Benefits:
> boosts body core strength; improves focus, balance, and memory; calms mind; relieves headache; strengthens spine

Equipment:
> yoga mat

Level:
> intermediate

Directions:
> I. On your yoga mat, go on all fours. Press your palms firmly into the ground.
> II. Gently raise your right leg, look up, and form an arch with your back.
> III. Inhale and exhale deeply through your nose.
> IV. Stay in position for about 10 seconds.

22. Half Moon Pose (or *Ardha Chandrasana*)

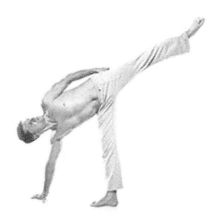

Benefits:
improves balance, blood circulation, and flexibility; relaxes liver and spleen; stretches leg muscles

Equipment:
yoga mat

Level:
intermediate

Directions:
I. On your yoga mat, stand straight.
II. Gently bend sideward while raising your left leg. Support yourself with your hands.
III. Inhale and exhale deeply through your nose.
IV. Stay in position for about 5 seconds.

23. Reverse Table Pose (or *Ardha Purvottanasana*)

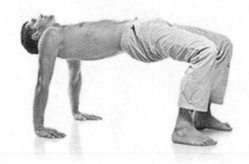

Benefits:
 improves focus, endurance; reduces stress; strengthens arms and legs

Equipment:
 yoga mat

Level:
 intermediate

Directions:
 I. On your yoga mat, sit down in a cross-legged position.
 II. Firmly place your hands behind you.
 III. Gently raise yourself as high as your arms can support you.
 IV. Inhale and exhale deeply through your nose.
 V. Stay in position for about 5 seconds.

24. Plank (or *Dandasana Chaturanga*)

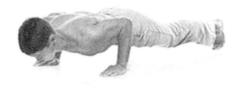

Benefits:

corrects posture; improves balance; improves the flexibility of legs; strengthens back and forearms

Equipment:

yoga mat

Level:

intermediate

Directions:

I. Lie gently with your face on the floor.

II. Align your hands to your chest. Make sure that your feet are straight.

III. Gently raise your body and allow your hands and feet to support your feet.

IV. Inhale and exhale deeply through your nose.

25. Seated Forward Bend (or *Paschimottasana*)

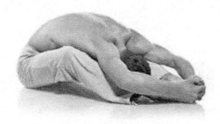

Benefits:

    corrects posture; improves the flexibility of legs; strengthens abdominal muscles, legs, and thighs

Equipment:

    yoga mat; yoga block

Level:

    intermediate

Directions:

    I. Sit down on your yoga mat

    II. Position your legs in front.

    III. You may use your yoga block to support back.

    IV. Extend body and arms forward; if possible, touch toes.

    V. Inhale and exhale deeply through your nose.

26. Frog Pose (or *Bhekasana*)

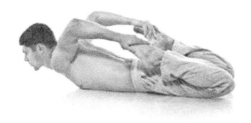

Benefits:

calms mind; corrects posture; reduces stress; strengthens back

Equipment:

yoga mat; yoga belt

Level:

intermediate

Directions:

I. On your yoga mat, lie on your belly.

II. You may use yoga belt for support. Slowly hold feet from the back.

III. Slowly raise chest and squeeze one shoulder toward the other shoulder.

IV. Around the hips, fold feet and hold toes with hands.

V. Inhale and exhale deeply through your nose.

27. Boat Poseanudocat (or *Halasanas*)

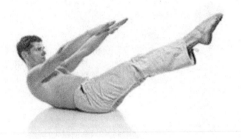

Benefits:
improves digestive function; reduces belly fat; regulates blood circulation; strengthens spine and hip muscles

Equipment:
yoga mat

Level:
intermediate

Directions:
I. In a seated position, bend your knees and place your feet firmly on the ground.
II. Gently lean back and raise your feet. Make sure that your spine is straight.
III. Gently raise your arms. Make sure that they are parallel to your raised feet.
IV. Inhale and exhale deeply through your nose.

28. Downward Dog (or *Adho Mukha Svanasana*)

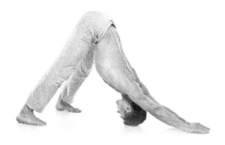

Benefits:

finds body balance; improves memory; strengthens the pelvic floor

Equipment:

yoga mat

Level:

intermediate

Directions:

I. On top of the yoga mat, stand straight.

II. Gently lower self by bending downward.

III. Inhale and exhale deeply through your nose.

Level III Yoga Poses

29. Standing Yoga Seal Pose (or *Dandayamana Yoga Mudrasana*)

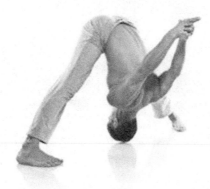

Benefits:
    improves blood circulation; relieves headache

Equipment:
    yoga mat

Level:
    Challenging

Directions:
    I. On your yoga mat, stand with feet wide apart.
    II. Gently bend down until your head reaches the ground.
    IV. Clasp your hands together at your back.
    V. Inhale and exhale deeply through your nose.
    VI. Stay in position for about 10 seconds.

30. Front Split Pose (or *Hanumanasana*)

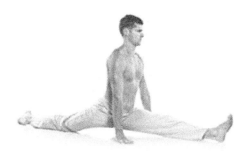

Benefits:

  eases ankle and knee injuries; improves balance and flexibility; strengthens inner thighs and legs

Equipment:

  yoga mat

Level:

  Challenging

Directions:

  I. On your yoga mat, gently perform a split.
  II. Support the position with each hand at the side.
  III. Inhale and exhale deeply through your nose.
  IV. Stay in position for about 5 seconds.

31. Extended Side Angle (or *Utthita Parsvakonasana*)

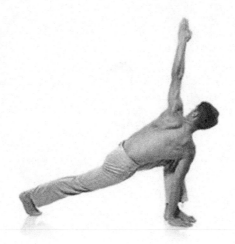

Benefits:
    improves balance, blood circulation, focus, and flexibility; relaxes liver and spleen; strengthens butt, hips, and thighs

Equipment:
    yoga mat

Level:
    Challenging

Directions:
    I. On your yoga mat, stand on your side.
    II. Perform a lunge.
    III. Gently twist your body.
    IV. Inhale through your nose. Raise one arm.
    V. Exhale through your nose. With the opposite arm, reach the ground.
    VI. Stay in position for about 5 seconds.

32. Triangle Pose (or *Utthita Trikanasana*)

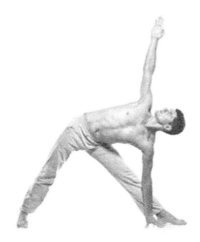

Benefits:

improves balance, blood circulation, and flexibility; relaxes liver and spleen; strengthens butt, hips, and thighs

Equipment:

yoga mat

Level:

Challenging

Directions:

I. On your yoga mat, stand with feet apart.

II. Form a triangle with your feet.

III. Gently bend your body and look upward.

IV. Inhale through your nose. Raise one arm.

V. Exhale through your nose. With the opposite arm, reach the ground.

VI. Stay in position for about 5 seconds.

33. Crescent Lunge (or *Anjanayesana*)

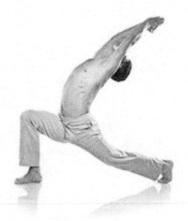

Benefits:
> corrects posture; improves balance, blood circulation, and focus; strengthens abdominal muscles, butt, hips, and thighs

Equipment:
> yoga mat

Level:
> Challenging

Directions:
> I. Stand on your side.
> II. Raise your arms.
> III. Perform a lunge.
> IV. Arch your back.
> V. Inhale and exhale deeply through your nose.
> VI. Stay in position for about 10 seconds.

34. Wide-Angle Standing Forward Bend (or *Prasarita Padottanasana*)

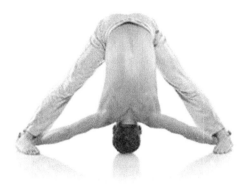

Benefits:

improves balance, blood circulation, focus, and memory; relieves headache

Equipment:

yoga mat

Level:

Challenging

Directions:

I. On your yoga mat, stand with feet wide apart.

II. Gently bend down until your head reaches the ground.

III. Inhale and exhale deeply through your nose.

IV. Secure the position by holding onto your ankles.

35. Supported Shoulder Stand (or *Salamba Sarvangasana*)

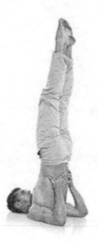

Benefits:
> improves balance and blood circulation; relieves headache; strengthens shoulders

Equipment:
> yoga mat

Level:
> Challenging

Directions:
> I. On your yoga mat, lie down.
> II. With the support of your hands, gently raise your body. Form a vertical line.
> III. Inhale and exhale deeply through your nose.

36. Simple Seated Twist (or *Bharadvaja*)

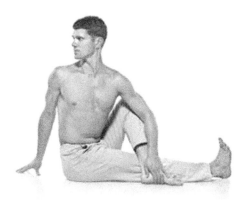

Benefits:
    calms mind; corrects posture; improves balance and flexibility; reduces stress; strengthens back, neck, and shoulders

Equipment:
    yoga mat

Level:
    Challenging

Directions:
    I. Sit straight on your yoga mat.
    II. Bring your legs in front of you.
    III. Gently swing your lower left leg over your right leg.
    IV. Support your stance with both arms. Support your left feet with your left hand. Meanwhile, place your right on the ground.
    V. Stay in position for about 10 seconds.
    VI. Inhale and exhale deeply through your nose.

37. Warrior Two Pose (or *Virabhadrasana*)

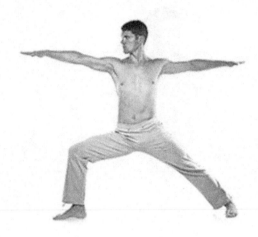

Benefits:
  calms mind; reduces stress; strengthens leg and lower body muscles

Equipment:
  yoga mat, yoga block

Level:
  Challenging

Directions:
  I. Stand straight on your yoga mat. Gently move each leg apart from the other. You may use your yoga block between your legs.
  II. Slowly twist right foot 90 degrees.
  III. Extend arms sideward; keep shoulders down and palms down.
  IV. Lunge into the left knee and form a 90-degree angle.
  V. Keep knee over foot; focus on maintaining position.
  VI. Inhale and exhale deeply through your nose.

38. Dancer Pose (or *Natarajasana*)

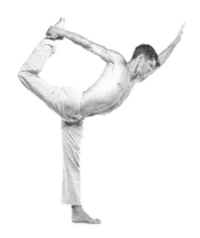

Benefits:

calms mind; corrects posture; improves balance and flexibility; reduces stress; strengthens back, neck, and shoulders

Equipment:

yoga mat

Level:

Challenging

Directions:

I. Stand straight.
II. Stretch one of your arms in front of you.
III. Raise your right leg and using your right arm, reach for it.
IV. Stay in position for about 10 seconds.
V. Inhale and exhale deeply through your nose.

39. Fish Pose (or *Matsyasan*)

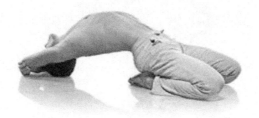

Benefits:
boosts energy; corrects posture; strengthens legs and back

Equipment:
yoga mat

Level:
Challenging

Directions:
I. Go into kneeling position and enclose your head inside your arms.
II. Gently bend to the ground until you are lying on your back. Make sure that your buttocks are resting on your soles.
III. Gently raise your abdominal muscles.
IV. Inhale and exhale deeply through your nose.

40. Extended Triangle Pose (or *Utthita Trikonasana*)

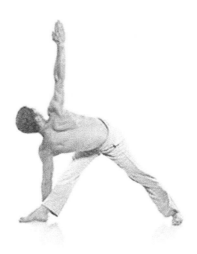

Benefits:

improves balance, concentration, and stability; strengthens arms and feet

Equipment:

yoga mat

Level:

Challenging

Directions:

I. On your yoga mat, stand with feet apart.

II. With left and right feet, form a 90-degree angle.

III. Modify formation into a triangle; with a 90-degree angle, use the ground as a base.

IV. Distribute weight evenly and extend arms sideward.

V. Raise toes with one arm and leave the other arm in the air.

VI. Inhale and exhale deeply through your nose.

Note: Always keep your mouth closed while you perform any of these techniques unless it is explicitly mentioned to do otherwise.

CHAPTER 4

YOGA SEQUENCES

In the previous chapter, you were introduced to different yoga poses for men– particularly, 20 poses. While it's all right to choose a random asana and match it with other random poses, as you chant "Om!" to form a sequence, it's recommended to choose poses accordingly. Doing so grants you better health benefits, as well as a satisfying yoga session.

Be Familiar with Different Yoga Sequences

Since you already learned the different asanas for men, it's time to take yoga practice sessions up a notch by becoming familiar with yoga sequences; you can also get around to the yoga sequences with a partner, which makes the habit even more fun. Basically, these are just certain poses that are accomplished in a certain order; they come with all the packaged benefits of each pose in the order. Although they can be tiring, performing the sequences regularly will benefit the physical and mental wellbeing.

Sequence # 1: Child's Pose – Forward Fold – Plough – Half-Fish - Frog

Sequence # 1 involves a lot of stretching and moving around (e.g. going into a standing position and going into a kneeling position); it's an ideal yoga sequence for men since, apart from the common physical and mental health perks, it comes with energy-boosting benefits.

Benefits:
> calms mind; corrects posture; improves the flexibility of thighs and arms, and back muscles; improves memory; reduces stress; strengthens back and pelvic floor

Time:

    10 minutes

Equipment:

    yoga mat; yoga belt

Level:

    easy

Directions:

1. Perform Child's Pose.
2. Go back to standing position and perform Forward Fold.
3. Slowly go into kneeling position and perform Plough.
4. Rest for 10-15 seconds and perform Half-Fish.
5. Slowly go back into kneeling position and perform Frog.

Sequence # 2: Hero Pose – Extended Triangle – Eagle – Down Dog – Seated Chest Lift

This yoga sequence is known to make you feel more confident while assisting in increasing the strength of the muscles in your legs, upper thighs, and chest. Although it can be performed any time of the day, it's best done in the mornings so you are granted the morale and physical boost at the start of your day; especially if you have a full schedule ahead of you, sparing not more than an hour for the exercise can give you necessary encouragement.

Benefits:

    calms mind; corrects posture; finds body balance; improves concentration and memory; improves the flexibility of back and legs; reduces stress; strengthens arms and feet, pelvic floor, and upper thighs

Time:

    10 minutes

Equipment:

    yoga mat, yoga block, and chair

Level:

    intermediate

Directions:

1. Perform *Hero Pose.*

2. Rest for 10-15 seconds. Then, go back to standing position and perform *Extended Triangle*.
3. Again, return to standing position and perform *Eagle*.
4. Rest for another 10-15 seconds before performing *Down Dog*.
5. Slowly get into the chair and perform *Seated Chest Lift*.

Sequence # 3: Standing Forward Bend – Seated Forward Bend – Puppy Pose – Thread & Needle – Warrior Pose

Yoga sequence # 3, although a bit complicated to get into during the second half of the sequence, is a powerful exercise since it keeps the mind occupied while working out the core muscles. If done regularly, the dudes can expect superior strength around the hip region. Other than that, eventually, they will notice a more relaxed presence.

Benefits:
    calms mind; corrects posture; improves the flexibility of legs; reduces stress; strengthens abdominal muscles, back, leg and lower body muscles neck, shoulders, and thighs

Time:
    20 minutes

Equipment:
    yoga mat, yoga block, and chair

Level:
    intermediate

Directions:
1. Perform *Standing Forward Bend*.
2. Rest for 10-15 seconds. Then, get on a chair and perform *Seated Forward Bend*.
3. Slowly return to standing position and perform *Puppy Pose*.
4. Rest for another 10-15 seconds and perform *Thread & Needle*.
5. Rest for yet another 10-15 seconds and perform *Warrior Pose*.

Sequence # 4: Dolphin – Crescent Lunge – Cobra – Bridge – Bow

This sequence is focused on eliminating stress; it involves more yoga poses that require lying down since the goal is to make you feel relaxed. If men are in search of a workout that can boost their concentration levels, this series of yoga poses are recommended.

Benefit:

> boosts energy; calms minds; finds body balance; improves endurance; improves the flexibility of legs, hips, thighs, and neck; improves memory; reduces stress; strengthens pelvic floor, feet, and shoulders

Time:

> 25 minutes

Equipment: yoga mat; yoga belt; yoga block

Level:

> Challenging

Directions:

1. Perform *Dolphin*.
2. Slowly go into standing position and perform *Crescent Lunge*.
3. Rest for 10-15 seconds and perform *Cobra*.
4. Gently lie down on the back and perform *Bridge*.
5. Slowly go back to standing position and perform *Bow*.

CHAPTER 5

CREATE & IMPLEMENT PERSONAL PLAN

Since you've learned the essentials in yoga for men, it's now time to create and implement your own yoga practice sessions. If you're just about to adopt this kind of workout, first, ask yourself whether you are willing to commit to yoga practice sessions for the long run; be honest so you could design a plan properly. For starters, a short plan will do the trick.

Create a Personal Yoga Routine

The final step in this book on yoga for men is to create a personal yoga routine. Be realistic and instead of adhering to a generalized yoga plan, make one based on your own lifestyle and preference.

By coming up with your own routine, you increase your chances of following through with yoga practice sessions. Given the fact that you're still at the beginning stage, you could be less prone to getting tired of the workouts if you were the one who selected each element in your plan.

Devising an Effective Yoga Plan

Devise a yoga routine that fits with your lifestyle, as well as your schedule; for instance, if you work a regular office job that requires a 9 to 5 attendance, create a plan based on this information. If the goal is to perform a batch of yoga workouts twice a day (i.e. once in the morning and once in the evening), make sure that you have enough time to accomplish the exercises.

Important reminders:

- Avoid disregarding physical conditions or any health issue. As mentioned, you need to be realistic; if unfit to perform certain poses, opt for others; this book covers 20 different yoga poses, and there are hundreds more that you're yet to discover

- Avoid the modification of certain asanas. In the event that you find them too challenging at your initial try, don't tweak them to fit your current abilities; instead, rely on gradual improvements. For instance, if a pose involves reaching for your toes, you should reach for your toes; you may be unable to have sufficient flexibility for the meantime, but eventually, you can improve.
- Choose yoga poses and yoga sequences accordingly; only include those that you're sure will work for your personality type. For instance, if you're the type who can get easily bored when lying down on your back, consider staying away from too many workouts that involve lying down

Sample 4-Week Yoga Plan

The sample 4-week yoga plan involves daily yoga practices of breathing techniques and yoga poses. Learn to set aside a few minutes every day; at the culmination of each week, you'll still perform breathing exercises, but instead of a particular yoga pose, a particular yoga sequence takes its place.

Week # 1

- Day 1: Practice Progressive Relaxation Breathing Technique + Bow (do this 5 times within the day)
- Day 2: Practice Kalapabhati Breathing Technique + Seated Forward Bend (do this 5 times within the day)
- Day 3: Practice Abdominal Breathing + Extended Triangle (do this 5 times within the day)
- Day 4: Practice Guided Visualization Breathing Technique + Bridge (do this 5 times within the day)
- Day 5: Practice Nadi Shodhana Breathing Technique + Thread & Needle (do this 5 times within the day)
- Day 6: Practice Drop and Arch Breathing Technique + Crescent Lunge (do this 5 times within the day)
- Day 7: Practice Alligator Breathing + Sequence # 1 (do this 5 times within the day)

Week # 2

- Day 8: Practice Equal Breathing + Standing Forward Bend (do this 5 times within the day)
- Day 9: Practice Intercostals Breathing Technique +Hero Post (do this 5 times within the day)
- Day 10: Practice Guided Visualization Breathing Technique + Dolphin (do this 5 times within the day)
- Day 11: Practice Alligator Breathing + Down Dog (do this 5 times within the day)
- Day 12: Practice Nadi Shodhana Breathing Technique + Eagle (do this 5 times within the day)
- Day 13: Practice Abdominal Breathing + Warrior Pose (do this 5 times within the day)
- Day 14: Practice Kalapabhati + Sequence # 2 (do this 2 times within the day)

Week # 3

- Day 15: Practice Breathe & Squeeze + Seated Chest Lift (do this 5 times within the day)
- Day 16: Practice Abdominal Breathing + Half-Fish (do this 5 times within the day)
- Day 17: Practice Drop and Arch Breathing Technique + Frog (do this 5 times within the day)
- Day 18: Practice Progressive Relaxation + Plough (do this 5 times within the day)
- Day 19: Practice Intercostals Breathing Technique + Eagle (do this 5 times within the day)
- Day 20: Practice Alligator Breathing + Crescent Lunge (do this 5 times within the day)
- Day 21: Practice Equal Breathing + Sequence # 3 (do this 2 times within the day)

Week # 4

- Day 22: Practice Guided Visualization Breathing Technique + Forward Fold (do this 5 times within the day)
- Day 23: Practice Nadi Shodhana Breathing Technique + Child's Pose (do this 5 times within the day)

- Day 24: Practice Alligator Breathing + Cobra (do this 5 times within the day)
- Day 25: Practice Abdominal Breathing + Extended Triangle (do this 5 times within the day)
- Day 26: Practice Equal Breathing + Dolphin (do this 5 times within the day)
- Day 27: Practice Progressive Relaxation Breathing Technique + Warrior Pose (do this 5 times within the day)
- Day 28: Practice Breathe & Squeeze + Sequence # 4 (do this 2 times within the day)

CHAPTER 6

HOW TO PRACTICE YOGA DAILY

It might not seem natural to include yoga into your daily routine. However, it does help to think about the different benefits just ten minutes of yoga offers. You can enhance your overall physical and mental health with yoga. If you can only set some time aside for yoga, it will be easy.

There are just two steps you have to follow to practice yoga daily. The first step is to incorporate yoga into your daily schedule. The second step is to vary your daily practice.

Step 1: Incorporate Yoga into Your Daily Schedule

Your yoga gear should be handy. If you want to practice yoga daily, then make sure that your yoga gear is always laid out. If you do this, then you won't be able to find any excuses not to do yoga daily. You need a yoga mat, maybe a yoga belt, blanket, and even a block. However, a simple yoga mat is sufficient for a beginner. You can buy the necessary yoga props from any sporting goods stores or also order it online. You don't need any specific yoga clothing per se. As long as your clothes are comfortable and don't constrain your movements, you are good to go. Anything that you can wear to the gym is suitable for yoga as well. Once you have all the necessary yoga gear, the next step is to decide when to practice and how long you want to practice.

There is no such thing as the perfect time to do yoga. However, if you want to include yoga in your daily schedule, then it is a good idea to practice it at the same time daily. It will help you to create a routine. You can practice it early in the morning if you are an early riser. Doing yoga, first thing in the morning will leave you feeling energized. Also, it will prevent you from making any excuses to skip yoga later in the day. You can practice it in the evening if you want to. It is better to create a routine. Once you fix a specific time to do yoga, it does get easy. Your body and mind will associate a particular time and place with your yoga session. Select a time slot wherein there wouldn't be any distractions or the distractions will be minimal, like early in the morning or late at night. You can practice yoga for as long as you want. It can be a couple of sets of Surya Namaskar (sun salutations) or even 90 minutes of the full session.

Set a specific time for yoga. Make sure that you turn off all the electronic gadgets, or at least put them on silent. Create a calm space for yourself without any distractions. Most of the yoga classes last for 60 to 95 minutes. You don't have to practice yoga in one go; you can even practice it in sets of ten minutes if you want to. The spot that you choose for yoga should be comfortable. It should be peaceful, should have soft lighting. It shouldn't be too cold or hot. You can even join a yoga class if you want to. If you have access to a garden, you can practice yoga in the garden. Regardless of where you want to practice yoga, the place should have room for plenty of movement.

You will experience a gradual change in your overall health when you practice yoga daily. The difference won't be overnight, and it does take a while. At times, you might even feel like you aren't progressing. Give it some time and be consistent in your efforts. You certainly will see a change. If you do miss one session of yoga, don't make a big deal of it. It is okay and continue from where you left off previously.

Step Two: Vary Your Daily Practice

The key is to be regular, not rigorous. It is better to practice yoga daily for a couple of minutes instead of a lengthy session on an irregular basis. Start with any asana you want to, but don't start with really complicated ones. Regardless of the pose that you want to begin with, perfect it before you move on to something else. It is okay to do some yoga instead of none and do remind yourself of this. Have a positive and not a negative mindset towards yoga. Don't worry if you don't get a pose correctly; try again. Don't tell yourself that you cannot do something. You certainly can do any pose, if you just practice a little. Practice yoga regularly and you can slowly move on to the more difficult ones.

The next step is to create a sequence of yoga poses to practice. It can be a challenging step, mainly if you practice yoga at home. Set up a different series that you can practice daily. The key is to get all the benefits of yoga without getting bored. If you practice the same sequence daily, you will end up getting bored. You can start the practice with meditation and some chanting exercises to clear your mind. It will also help you to focus your thoughts. Before you begin to practice, think about the reasons that motivate you. If you cannot think of a specific purpose, try going through the list of advantages yoga offers. Then you can move onto to warm up exercises like the Surya Namaskar. Always end your yoga session with something that relaxes you. Design your yoga schedule in such a manner that it contains easy and challenging poses.

It is entirely reasonable that you wouldn't be able to do all the yoga asanas every day. You can incorporate poses from all the types of asanas into your daily schedule so that it doesn't bore you. Start with the asanas that are easy, and you can slowly move onto the poses that are more difficult. Perform poses from each of the asanas in this order: Standing poses, inversions, then the backbends, and at last the forward bends. To elevate the stress on your spine between the backbends and the forward bends, add a twisting asana. You should be able to hold each of the asanas for at least 3 to 5 breaths. Always end your yoga session with the corpse pose. It will relax your body and calm your mind as well.

If you like to chant mantras before or after your yoga session, then do so. However, make sure that you change the chant daily. There are different mantras that you can use, and each of these mantras tends to correspond with your intention. The repetition of a mantra will distract you from the stress you feel, and it will also help to maintain your focus. The most basic mantra is Om or Aum. It is quite powerful and chanting this mantra will fill your body with positive vibrations. It is usually combined with the "Shanti" mantra. Shanti in Sanskrit means peace. You can repeat Om as many times as you want to. There is another mantra that's known as the maha-mantra. The maha or the great mantra is to chant "Hare Krishna." It usually helps to bring you mental peace. You just have to keep repeating the words "Hare Krishna" over and over again. Another mantra that you can chant is "Lokah samastha sukhino bhavantu." This mantra helps to foster happiness and freedom.

Repeat this mantra thrice or even more than that if you want to. The mantras that you chant in yoga have one purpose, to calm your mind and bring you peace. It is quite easy to incorporate yoga into your daily schedule. All that matters is whether you want to do it daily or not.

CHAPTER 7

TIPS FOR BEGINNERS

Yoga is a brilliant form of exercise. Regardless of whether you are doing yoga for the first time, or are a yoga veteran, the joy that comes from yoga is the same. You might even experience more joy than the experienced ones. However, it is quite likely that you will run into a couple of pesky obstacles along the way. For instance, the vocabulary of yoga might be a little challenging to get the hang of. Sanskrit does sound exotic, but the western eyes might glaze over rather quickly. If someone asked you to read "pashchimottanasana," you might stumble a little. Another problem that you might run into is with the execution of yoga asanas. Don't worry even if an asana sounds absurd. It is designed for a specific purpose. Will I be sitting like that and will I be comfortable as well? Well, you will be! Maybe not immediately, but you certainly will after a while. All beginners need a little empathy.

The most difficult challenge that you might face as a beginner is to create a yoga practice at home. For that, you have to select a list of techniques and arrange them into a schedule. There are different practices that you will learn, not immediately, but at least eventually you will. Another question that might bother you is "Is it important?" Well, all the yoga poses are essential. Each pose has a specific effect on the part of the human body. In this section, you will learn about specific tips that a beginner can use. Most of these tips are practical, and the rest encourage you to develop a positive mindset. However, one thing that's common for all these tips is that they call for action. It doesn't make any sense if you just read these tips and leave it at that. So, go through this chapter carefully and start to practice these tips as well. Let us get started now.

Maintain a journal

A yoga session always constitutes several comments and insights that help to smoothen out the rough edges of life. It can even change the way you perceive yourself and the world around you. However, today's "aha" moment is often forgotten in the thoughts of tomorrow's activities. So, make a note of it. Write down your feelings and experiences about the yoga practice in a journal. You merely need to write your observations and insights in your notebook. It might sound a little old school, but it is efficiently quoted. Make a list of all the poses you practice along with the new ones that you learn. List any new terms that you learn as well. If you have any questions while you meditate, make a note of it as well. The idea is to journalize all that you feel while you practice yoga. You never know, a brilliant idea might strike you when you do this.

Be "artsy"

If you find it difficult to remember all that you have to do in a particular pose, you can draw it. Simple stick figures can help you to retain the necessary information about a posture. Let your inner artist come to the forefront. Use arrows to mark the movements in a pose. When you do this once, the position will be etched into your memory. It is also a great way to recollect all that you did in the yoga practice session. If you want, you can download the pictures of the poses from the Internet and create your yoga scrapbook. Well, it is up to you. The idea is to remember the yoga postures so that you don't have to keep checking what needs to be done while you practice yoga.

Make some space

If you want to practice yoga at home, then you have to make sure that you have a designated spot to do yoga. Create a Zen den for your yoga practice. Select a room with the least amount of distractions and store all your yoga props in it. You can even get an oriental rug or place some images or statues that have a calming effect on the mind. The idea is to create a sacred space where your mind can relax and unwind. You cannot practice yoga with loud music blaring in the background.

Define your practice

The yoga routine that you create solely depends on you. You should define the time that you can allocate towards the practice of yoga. Not just that, you should also decide the technique you want to focus and the balance that you want to strike between meditation, breathing exercises and the practice of asanas. If you aren't sure how to go about it, then consider a couple of details. Do you understand the order of the methods you use and your practice? Are there any particular aspects of an asana that you need to focus on? Do you need to learn more about any asanas you use? If a specific pose seems too complicated for you, can you simplify it? Is it possible to break down the aspects of an asana? What are the steps that you are good at? What are the different methods of relaxation and meditation that you learned? If you have any doubts about any of these questions, please refer to the relevant chapters in this book! All the information that you need to practice yoga is mentioned within the pages of this book.

A good sticky mat

It might seem like a trivial detail - however, you can never underestimate the importance of sound footing. If you have never used a yoga mat, you can perhaps borrow one and see for yourself. Or you can go to any of the sporting goods stores and try out a couple of yoga mats. Your mat should provide you a good grip when you perform any poses that require you to stretch your legs or your torso. Once you try a mat, you will understand whether it is a good fit for you or not.

Balance is important

Yoga isn't just about the practice of different postures. You need to include positions and relaxation techniques into your yoga routine. It is essential to strike a good balance between these two aspects of yoga. You cannot neglect one to concentrate on the other. Some might want to focus on the meditational aspects of yoga while others might like the physical health benefits it offers. However, you need to understand that the idea of yoga is to enhance your physical and mental health. You need to create that equilibrium in your yoga practice sessions.

Build a small library

Yoga videos can simplify your life. They teach you how to perform a pose. Not just that, stock up on a couple of yoga CDs as well as books. There is no such thing as too much knowledge. You can even play audio recordings to guide yourself through different poses.

Learn a little Sanskrit

If you like to learn new languages, then you can learn a couple of Sanskrit words. It is an elegant language and has a lot of technical names. All the yoga poses and techniques have Sanskrit names. It is a good idea to familiarize yourself with the different yoga jargon. It is quite an orderly language. Once you are comfortable with the basic pronunciations, you no longer have to mumble the words. Most of the syllables in Sanskrit tend to begin with a consonant and then end with a vowel. The letters in Sanskrit have fixed pronunciations, unlike English. So, once you know how to pronounce the letters in Sanskrit, you can quickly master different words. If you can correctly pronounce the words used in a Sanskrit mantra, the effect it has will be better.

Breathing breaks

You can efficiently manage your stress through breathing exercises. You can use breath awareness to diffuse a moment of anxiety, panic, or even fear. However, you should think about extending these breathing breaks and use them somewhat regularly. When you use these breaks frequently, also if it is only for a couple of minutes at a time, you will notice a positive change in your mindset. You will get better at managing your stress. During your work hours, take a break for a couple of minutes. Whenever you take a break, close your eyes and concentrate on your breathing. Count the number of breaths you take. It will help you to overcome any stress that's building up in your body. Not just that, it relaxes your respiratory muscles as well. Make sure that you include simple breathing exercises into your daily routine.

Let the posture do its work

You might feel like you should do something while you perform a pose or an exercise. Yes, you do have to put the necessary effort to master a pose. However, at times all you need to do is sit back and let the exercise do its work. While you perform a breathing exercise, you have to concentrate on your breath essentially. There is nothing else that you have to do. So, instead of thinking that you aren't doing anything, just enjoy the exercise you perform. No effort is as bad as too much effort, and neither is desirable. So, the next time you perform the corpse pose, merely let the posture do its work for you.

Sleep is critical

The idea of waking up early to perform yoga, then have a good breakfast, and a quick stroll around the block does sound good, doesn't it? However, it will just stay an idea if you burn yourself out. If your body doesn't get sufficient rest, it cannot perform all that you want it to. You cannot wake up early if you keep going to bed late at night. Make sure that you get at least 7 hours of undisturbed sleep every night. It is okay to stay until daybreak once in a while. However, you shouldn't become habitually nocturnal. Without the necessary rest, you cannot feel better. After all, your body isn't a tireless machine.

Shush the critics

All those voices in your head that say you haven't accomplished anything or the ones that say that yoga isn't helpful should be ignored. Ignore all the cynics that rest within your mind. You cannot expect to derive the benefits of yoga overnight. Practice yoga consistently for at least three weeks before you jump to any conclusions about whether it does you any good or not. Learn to appreciate this process; only then can you reap the benefits it offers.

CHAPTER 8

YOGA POSES FOR SEXUAL HEALTH

Yoga can improve your sexual health. In this chapter, you will learn about the different yoga poses that will enhance your sexual health.

Butterfly Pose

Place your mat on the floor. Sit down on the mat and make sure that your back is straight. Now, bend your knees so that the soles of your feet are pressed together. Place them as close to your crotch as you can. Initially, your knees might not touch the floor, and that's okay. Hold the butterfly pose and focus on your inner thighs. Push down on your knees so that they are as close to the floor as they possibly can be. You will feel slight tension in your thigh muscles when you perform this pose. Relax, it happens and it's natural. You can close your eyes to improve your focus.

Hold this pose for three minutes. It helps to tone the channels of sexual energy and also your reproductive organs.

Seated forward bend

Place the mat on the floor. Sit down on the mat and keep your back straight. Stretch your legs in front of you. Now lean forward and move your arms towards your toes. Let your knees stretch ahead and don't lock them. Allow your upper torso to relax and feel the slight stretch in your back and the back of your legs. However, don't overstretch your body, or you will hurt yourself. Take long and deep breaths through your nostrils. If you are flexible, then you can even grab your shins, ankles, or toes (if you are incredibly limber). Hold this pose for a minute. Then slowly return to your original position. Repeat this pose three times in a session. If you want to increase your mobility, then this is a good pose, and it also helps to stimulate the sexual energy in your body.

Chair Pose

As the name suggests, you have to mimic the pose of sitting in a chair, sans the chair. It isn't difficult! You use your thigh muscles to hold the pose. While you do this, you have to keep your arms pointing upwards, near your ears. Keep your legs squeezed together, for better balance. Hold this position for fifteen seconds. You can even modify it and hold it for longer, but that depends on your strength and endurance. Repeat this exercise thrice, and you can work your way towards ten reps. It not only strengthens the muscles in your leg but also facilitates the movement of your sexual energy to your energy centers.

Runner's Stretch

The runner's stretch is just a fancy name for a lunge. You have to stand straight on the yoga mat, and then place your right leg forward a few feet. When you do this, bend your right knee and keep your left leg stretched out straight. Do not allow your knee to go past your ankle when you stretch. You can either place your hands on your hips or put them on either side of your right foot for better support. You will feel the muscles in your left leg stretch, and it strengthens your right leg. Hold this pose to the count of ten deep and slow breaths. Once you do this, return to the standing posture on your mat. Now, repeat the same with your other leg. This position helps to strengthen your pelvic floor muscles, improves your flexibility, as well as stamina.

Cobra Pose

The cobra pose is not just good for your sexual health, but it helps with any lower back pain that you experience. It also helps to correct your posture. Place yourself on all fours, and your arms should be shoulder width apart, while your knees are almost touching. You have to slowly lower your body while you keep your upper torso elevated. Keep your arms straight, and your elbows should point towards your body. You can look upwards, provided you don't have any neck issues. You can rest on your forearms if you feel any discomfort in your lower back or abdomen. The basic idea is to imitate the pose of a cobra when it is ready to strike. Initially, hold this pose for 30 seconds, and you can increase it slowly to three minutes. It stimulates your sexual centers of energy to enhance your performance and vitality.

Sat Kriya pose

Sit on the heels of your feet or on your feet and keep your knees bent. If you feel that's difficult, just kneel down. You can even place a towel under your knees for additional padding. Now, slowly stretch your arms above your head. Your elbows should be close to your head. If that's not comfortable for you, merely stretch your arms upwards as high as possible. Intertwine all your fingers apart from the index fingers. Your index fingers should point upwards in a straight angle. Cross one thumb over the other. Shut your eyes and start the following set of contractions. If you want to, you can say "sat" whenever you inhale and "kriya" when you exhale. You have to inhale and exhale through your nose and close your mouth. You will notice that your abdominal muscles will contract and it all starts from your navel. Inhale through your nose and contract the muscles around your stomach. You will feel slight contractions in the muscles around your navel, rectum, and your groin. It is known as "root" lock. Hold your breath in for a moment; visualize the movement of energy from your buttocks, along the length of your spine to your head. Exhale through your nose slowly, release the root lock, and then do it twice. Rest for a couple of seconds and repeat the exercise. You should do this exercise for at least three minutes, and you can slowly work your way towards ten minutes. If your limbs feel tired, take a break for a couple of seconds. However, try to do this for at least three minutes. It is a beneficial pose to tone your sexual organs, and it helps with any sexual dysfunction as well.

Frog Pose

To start this pose, you have to squat on your toes. Place your feet apart while your heels are pressed together. Lift your arms to gain better balance. Breathe in through your nose and stand up while you lower your head towards your knees. Start to lower your heels as you stand up straight. Make sure that your fingers touch the floor. It is okay if you aren't able to straighten your legs fully. Now, slowly exhale through your nose. You have completed one rep of this exercise. Inhale as you start the next rep while you return to the squatting position. You can gradually work your way up to ten reps of the frog pose. Of course, you can do more reps if your body permits. It might sound deceptively simple, but it does take a lot of effort. Don't hold your breath in and breathe slowly.

It is an excellent pose to improve your sexual health, tone the muscles in your leg and speed up your heart rate. If you have any issues with your knees, you should skip this exercise. If you don't have any knee trouble, then please go ahead. However, stop whenever your knees hurt. You can suffer from hemorrhoids if you do too many reps of the frog pose. Also, take a break whenever you start to feel dizzy or lightheaded.

Plough Pose

Lie down on the yoga mat. Now, start to draw your knees towards your chest. Roll backward and let your legs extend way past your head. Stretch your legs as much as you can. You can support your back with your hands. In this pose, your toes should touch the ground. Well, it will take you a while to get there. If you are quite limber, then you can do this pose easily. You should feel the muscles in your leg stretch and some contraction in your abdomen. Don't overdo it or else you can seriously hurt your back. Take in long and deep breaths. Hold this pose for anywhere between 1 to 3 minutes. If you feel dizzy or lightheaded, stop immediately.

It is a great position to enhance your sexual system. However, for a beginner, it is a good idea to take it slow. Make sure that you don't put any unnecessary strain on the muscles in your back, neck, and hamstrings.

Rock pose

It is a relaxing and straightforward pose for your body. Place yourself on the edge of your yoga mat and tuck yourself into a ball. Your knees should be bent towards your chest and wrap your arms around your shins. You mainly have to curl up into a ball. Breathe like you usually do and rock onto your back. Once you rock onto your back, roll back again to a seated pose. Don't roll onto your neck, or you can hurt yourself gravely. Continue to roll like a ball for thirty seconds and work your way towards a minute.

This pose helps to strengthen your core and stimulate the centers of sexual energy in your body.

The Bridge Pose

Lie down on the yoga mat and place your feet as close to your butt as you possibly can while your knees are bent. Gently lift your torso upwards while you press down with your feet. Tighten the muscles in your thighs and buttocks. Lift your navel off the ground as high as you can. Hold the bridge for at least thirty seconds and slowly work your way towards three minutes. It is a powerful position. When you complete a set, gradually lower your back onto the yoga mat, one vertebra at a time. Lower yourself until you are lying on the mat with your knees bent. Repeat this exercise thrice. It helps to strengthen your pelvic muscles, and it also enhances your core and legs. You can feel the sexual energy move through your body from the base of your spine to your head.

Corpse Pose

Well, the corpse pose is the easiest yoga asana there is. As the name suggests, you only have to lie down on your yoga mat like a corpse. Close your eyes and place your hands on either side of your body. Breathe regularly and don't let any worries distract you. Inhale and exhale through your nose. The Shavasana or the corpse pose is the best way to end your yoga session. If you like listening to music, then play some soothing music. You can do this for up to 11 minutes.

If you want to improve your sexual health, then these positions will undoubtedly come in handy.

CHAPTER 9

YOGA MEDITATION

Yoga is a Sanskrit word that means union with the cosmos or divine energy. It involves various stretching exercises, and it has been around for thousands of years. Well, by now you know the history of yoga and the multiple benefits it offers.

If you want to practice yoga meditation, there are three steps that you have to follow. The first step is to create an environment that's conducive for mediation. The second step is to perform the basic poses. The third step is to focus on your mind and soul.

Create a meditation spot

The first step is to create a quiet environment. Select a place that is free of clutter and loud noises. You should feel comfortable if you want to practice yoga or meditation. If the spot is too noisy, then you cannot concentrate, especially if you are a beginner. An ideal location should be devoid of all electronic gadgets. Or find a place where you can block all the external sounds. It will be helpful if you can find a room where natural light filters in through the windows. If not, the lighting should be soft and not too harsh. Flickering lights are obviously a distraction, aren't they? Select a room with some natural heat, light, and air. It is not just the sounds that are a distraction; even machinery can be quite uncomfortable.

If you cannot do yoga or meditate in the open, find a place that has some radiant heat. Create cross ventilation by opening a door or a window. Let some fresh air into the room. If your tummy is full, you will relax too much, and it will make you drowsy. At the same time, if your yoga or meditation session is too close to mealtime, your hunger pangs can be quite distracting. Perhaps you can practice meditation a couple of hours before your mealtime, or a couple of hours after your meal. If not, you can always have a light snack before you start to meditate. It is essential to provide your body with the necessary sustenance to keep it functioning. Before you begin to meditate or perform yoga, you should do some light stretching or warm-up exercises. Warm up exercises will get the blood pumping in your body and will make you feel relaxed. Not just that, your concentration will also improve while you meditate. If your body feels limber, then you can sit for longer. Concentrate on your back and your core for a couple of minutes. Simple twists and bends will do the trick. You can practice Sukshma yoga before you meditate. For sukshma yoga, you have to gently squeeze your eyebrows a couple of times using your fingers. Roll your eyes a couple of times. Then rub your jawline as well as your temples to relax your facial muscles. Grab your ears and slowly tug them downwards.

Perform meditative poses

For starters, sit upright. You can rest on any surface you want, as long as it allows you to sit correctly. You can sit on the floor or the chair. Don't make your body rigid and let it be limber. Sitting cross-legged while you meditate is quite common. However, that's not the only way to relax. You can alternate the leg that rests on top while you meditate. Being comfortable is the main point. For better spinal alignment, you can gently tug on your chin.

Once you find a comfortable spot for yourself and have settled in, the next step is to follow the techniques of deep breathing. Focus on your breath and nothing else. You can just count the number of times you inhale and exhale through your nose. Or you can even perform nadi shodan. Nadi shodan is a technique of pranayama. Lift your right hand so that your thumb, little finger and ring finger are pointing outwards while the rest curl inwards. To close your right nostril, place your thumb gently on it and inhale through the left one. Once you inhale, you have to close the left nostril with your ring and little finger. Only after you close your left nostril, you can exhale through the right one. After you exhale through the right nostril, inhale through the same one. To exhale, you have to close the right nostril and let go of your breath through the left one. Once you do this with your right nostril, repeat the same steps with your left nostril.

Another breathing exercise that you can practice for meditating is to perform Samasthiti. The pose of Samasthiti is quite similar to the pose of an army person standing at attention. You have to be mindful of your balance and steadiness. Once you stand at attention, join your palms together (like you would when you pray). Breathe in slowly and raise your hands over your head. When you start to exhale, return your hands to your chest. Do this exercise for two minutes to calm your mind.

The next exercise that you can do is to perform the cow pose. Get on all fours and place your palms under your shoulders to support yourself. Breathe in deeply and raise your head along with your upper torso. While you elevate your upper body, lower your spine slowly towards the floor. You are mostly pushing your spine closer to your stomach. Complete this position by returning to a perfectly aligned back while you exhale.

The next asana you can perform to meditate is Vajrasana. To perform Vajrasana, you have to assume a sitting position. Once you do that, place your hands on the side and move your left foot so that it is in contact with your left buttock. Repeat the same with your right foot. Once you do this, you will be in a squatting position. You can lean forward and shift your body weight onto your knees. Lean backward into the space available between your heels. Breathe like you usually do for a couple of minutes. At the end of this pose, your toes should be touching one another. Make sure that you keep your core coiled to encourage better posture. Your body should be upright while you perform this pose.

The last meditative yoga exercise you can perform is the ujjayi breathing. Ujjayi breath is a long and smooth breath. It will not only calm you down but will make you feel quite energetic as well. You have to sit cross-legged on the floor. Try to relax your body and mind. Imagine that you are taking in deep and slow breaths (like breathing through a straw). Now exhale slowly (through the same imaginary straw). Make your breathing as slow and deliberate as you possibly can.

Focus on your body, mind, and soul

Forget about all the distractions. Don't think about any of your daily stresses and worries. The first step of meditation yoga is to embrace all the different things that go on in your life. Acknowledge all the chaos that you feel. You cannot only ignore your worries. Instead, embrace them and accept it all. After all, you are just a human being and worries are a significant part of human nature. Only when you recognize all the distractions, can you move beyond them and focus on yourself. Instead, concentrate on your body. Focus your attention inwards, towards the base of your spine. Focus your attention on the center of your body, to your spinal column and all the different parts of your body. Take stock of all the different parts of your body and all your different senses. Acknowledge all that you feel and think. Think about how your body functions and how each of the different parts functions like a well-oiled machine. Notice if you feel any pain or discomfort. If you want to reach a higher level of concentration while you meditate, you should will your mind to become silent. You have to set your mind at ease, and you can do so by concentrating on your breathing. If you want to become aware of your mind, then you should follow the four functions of the mind. The four functions of the mind are to observe, accept, understand, and train. You have to see all the impressions present in your mind like ego, judgments, or any prejudices. The next step is to accept all the observations you have without being critical of them. Forget about whether a particular observation is good or bad, and don't berate yourself for it. The next step is to understand your thought process. The way your mind functions and discerns things. The final step is to train your mind. You need to realize that you are in complete control of your mind and it isn't the other way around. You should train your consciousness.

Once you do this, the next step is to focus on a single object. If you have just started with meditation, during the initial phases, it might be difficult for you to concentrate fully. It is quite likely that your attention will lapse. Whenever you feel like your attention sways, you should redirect it towards a specific object. Try to focus on a single item. Like a piece of floorboard, a spot on the wall, or even a stationary object. At the end of your meditation session, you should bring your mind to attention. Take charge of your mind and be aware of all the small changes in your body. You can lightly ball your fists for a couple of minutes. Alternatively, you can even flex the muscles in your calf. A simple way to focus on your muscles is by smiling.

CHAPTER 10

SURYA NAMASKAR

One of the most beneficial yoga practices is that of Surya Namaskar. Surya Namaskar means sun salutation. The Sanskrit word for sun is Surya and Namaskar implies salutation. It is a way to greet the sun god and honor it. Surya Namaskars helps to cleanse your mind, body, as well as the soul. The ideal time to practice Surya Namaskars is early in the morning with an empty stomach. It engages all the different parts of your body and makes use of a couple of breathing techniques as well. It has plenty of benefits like it improves the health of your cardiovascular and digestive systems. Not just that, it improves your overall flexibility as well. There are twelve asanas included in this exercise, and you will learn about them in this chapter. Ideally, you should perform Surya Namaskars 108 times. However, as a beginner, you can start with 20 reps and increase the number as you progress.

Stage 1. Pranamasana

It is also known as the Prayer Pose. Stand at the edge of your mat with your legs placed close together. Inhale through your nose as you lift your arms above your head. Now exhale slowly through your nose and bring your palms together (like you are praying), and place them in front of your chest. It should seem like you are praying.

Stage 2. Hasta Uttansana

It is also known as the Raised Arms Pose. Inhale through your nose and lift your arms up and slowly move them backward. When you do this, ensure that your biceps are close to your ears. The goal is to stretch your body.

Stage 3. Hastapaadasana

It is also known as the Hand to Foot Pose. Exhale through your nose and bend your body forward while your palms face downward and your fingertips are aligned with your toes. Bow your knees slightly if you feel any discomfort. It is a forward bend and nothing else. It does get more comfortable with time, and you can perform this pose even when your legs are kept straight. Now, slowly exhale and bring your hands towards the floor. Try and see if you can touch your feet.

The name of this pose is the combination of two Sanskrit words. Hasta means hands and padah or pada means foot. So, this position is about making your hands meet your feet, quite literally. It helps to strengthen your back muscles and make your body limber.

Stage 4. Ashwa Sanchalanasana

It is also known as the Equestrian Pose. Once you complete the previous level, you have to inhale and push your left leg back slowly. Stretch it as far as you can. Now, bring the right foot forward, and you should place your foot between your hands.

Stage 5. Kumbhakasana

It is also known as the Plank Pose. Don't exhale after the previous step and stretch your left leg backward slowly. Support your bodyweight with the help of your toes and hands. Now, your body will be perfectly aligned, and the position resembles that of a plank and hence the name.

Stage 6. Ashtanga Namaskara

It is also known as the Salute with 8 Parts. Now, slowly move your knees towards the floor while you exhale. Slightly bend your knees towards the floor. Lower your chest and chin towards the floor. So, eight parts of your body will touch the floor. The eight parts are your knees, chin, hands, chest, and feet.

Stage 7. Bhujangasana

It is also known as the Cobra Pose. Well, you know how to perform the cobra pose by now. Here is a quick recap. Place yourself on all fours, and your arms should be shoulder width apart, while your knees are almost touching. You have to slowly lower your body while you keep your upper torso elevated. Keep your arms straight, and your elbows should point towards your body. You can look upwards, provided you don't have any neck issues. You can rest on your forearms if you feel any discomfort in your lower back or abdomen.

Stage 8. Adho Mukha Svanasana

It is also known as the Downward Facing Dog Pose. Exhale slowly through your nose after the seventh step and curl up your toes. Slowly raise your hips and pivot them so that your body forms the shape of an inverted V. Now, push your heels outward while you keep your head down. Arch your shoulders back. After this step, you will repeat the first four steps in the reverse order.

Stage 9. Ashwa Sanchalanasana

It is also known as the Equestrian Pose. Once you complete the previous step, you have to slowly inhale and push your left leg back. Stretch it as far as you can. Now, bring the right foot, and you should place your foot between your hands.

Stage 10. Hastapaadasana

It is also known as the Hand to Foot Pose. Exhale through your nose and bend your body forward while your palms face downward and your fingertips are aligned with your toes. Bend your knees slightly if you feel any discomfort. It is a forward bend and nothing else. It does get more comfortable with time, and you can perform this pose even when your legs are kept straight. Now, slowly exhale and bring your hands towards the floor. Try and see if you can touch your feet.

Stage 11. Hasta Uttansana

It is also known as the Raised Arms Pose. Inhale through your nose and lift your arms up and slowly move them backward. When you do this, ensure that your biceps are close to your ears. The goal is to stretch your body.

Stage 12. Pranamasana

It is also known as the Prayer Pose. Stand at the edge of your mat with your legs placed close together. Inhale through your nose as you lift your arms above your head. Now, exhale slowly through your nose and bring your palms together (like you are praying), and place them in front of your chest.

Now that you are familiar with all the twelve steps of Surya Namaskar, the next step is to practice it.

CONCLUSION

Thank you again for reading this book!

I hope this book was able to help you to learn about yoga for men. Hopefully, it's now clear to you that the practice is linked to a lineup of health benefits for the body and mind.

The next step is to design your own yoga routine. Since this book provides all the essentials, you can use it as a reference to incorporate yoga into your life. Surprise your peers; prove to them that you're man enough for yoga!

Finally, if you enjoyed this book, then I'd like to ask you for a favor, would you be kind enough to leave a review for this book on Amazon? I would **really appreciate it!**

Simply go to **bit.ly/YogaBookReview** to leave a review for this book on Amazon.

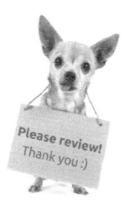

I would love for you to connect with me on Social Media with any questions, comments or just to experience beautiful images and inspirational quotes.

Amazing Instagram: **@Yogitation**

Website: www.qualitychapters.com

Thank you and good luck,
Michael Williams

DON'T FORGET TO GET
YOUR FREE BONUS GIFT!

Thanks again for taking your time to read my book. I would also like for you to continue on your path to a more peaceful and enjoyable life, therefore I'm going to give you the **"Yoga For All: The Simple Guide To Yoga & Meditation"** e-book for FREE!

Go to **bit.ly/freebookyoga** to download the FREE e-book.

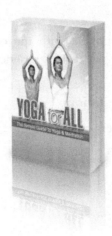

Preview of:

Mindfulness for Beginners: How to Live in The Present, Stress, and Anxiety Free

INTRODUCTION

Life is full of stress, and these days, it's so easy to fall into the traps of depression and anxiety. When that happens, you might feel like your life right now isn't good at all—and that you'd rather go back to the past because it's where your happiness lies.

That way of thinking is wrong. In fact, there are so many things you could do to help you forget about your worries, live in the present, and let go of anxiety and stress. You can start taking care of your mind— and mindfulness is a good start.

By reading this book, you will learn more about mindfulness, understand what mindfulness is about, why it's important, why eating and drinking slowly is important, how you can live a life free of stress and anxiety—and so much more!

Read this book now and find out how.

CHAPTER 1

WHAT MINDFULNESS IS AND WHAT IT IS NOT

Before anything else, what is mindfulness really about? And what it is not?

Mindfulness is...

To put it simply, mindfulness is about focusing on one's thoughts, emotions, and sensations without judgment, with intent, and with full acceptance. It has Buddhist roots, most especially Sati, which is part of the 7 Factors of Enlightenment. According to tradition, Sati is a way to recognize the dhammas, which are both reality and phenomena. When this is achieved, a person is well on his way to Nirvana, or a state of total serenity and happiness.

It was then popularized in America and other parts of the world by Jon Kabat-Zinn, the creator of the Stress Reduction Clinic, and a well-known Professor Emeritus. He then created the Mindfulness-Based Stress Reduction Technique, which aims to help people recognize their problems, not to wallow in them, but to actually exorcise them from their lives. Mindfulness is then believed to have a lot to do with the reduction of stress and anxiety.

In fact, a number of psychological and psychiatric facilities all over the world have been developing various techniques of mindfulness to help people undergoing therapy. In a way, they believe that science and meditation could actually go together, and bring some good in the world.

Clinical psychologists have said that the main reason why mindfulness is beneficial is because of the so-called two-component model. The said model is all about:

Self-Regulation, or how a person gets to control his attentiveness and gets to focus attention on his immediate experiences, so that it would be easy for him to live in the moment, and;

Adapting particular attention towards one's experiences, which would then help a person become more accepting, open, and curious.

When these work together, the person becomes whole—and so stress no longer would rule over his life.

However, it is not something that you should do to "escape" your life. It is more of connecting with your inner self. In short, it's about getting to know who you are, and not forgetting who you are.

It's also not about what you think, but rather about being self-aware and understanding of what's getting in and out of your head. It's also not about just one kind of experience alone. In fact, there are various mindfulness exercises that you can do—and that's what makes it useful.

Well, you also should keep in mind that mindfulness is not about becoming someone else, and not about becoming "perfect", but rather becoming who you truly are. Mindfulness helps you get into a right place—especially in your mind so you can apply calmness in your life.

And most importantly, mindfulness is not a religious practice. You can be part of any religion and you can enjoy the benefits of mindfulness. As aforementioned, it's really about getting to know yourself more—so you can harness your potential, and maximize its use in your life.

To check out the rest of the book, simply search for the title below on Amazon or go to: **bit.ly/Mindfulness4Beginners**

- *__Mindfulness for Beginners__ - How to Live in The Present, Stress, and Anxiety Free*

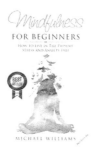

Thank you and good luck on your Yoga Journey!

Check Out My Other Books

Below you'll find my other books that are popular on Amazon and Kindle as well. Simply enter the name of the books in the search bar on Amazon to check them out. Alternatively, you can visit my author page on Amazon to see other work done by me.

For my authorpage, go to: **bit.ly/AuthorWilliams**

- ***Buddhism***: *Beginner's Guide to Understanding & Practicing Buddhism to Become Stress and Anxiety Free*

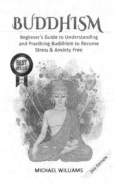

- ***Buddhism For Beginners*** *- How To Go From Beginner To Monk And Master Your Mind*

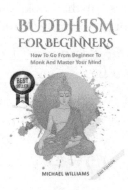

- ***Chakras For Beginners*** *– How to Awaken And Balance Chakras, Radiate Positive Energy And Heal Yourself*

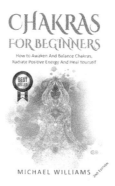

- ***Chakras for Beginners*** *- Awaken Your Internal Energy and Learn to Radiate Positive Energy and Start Healing*

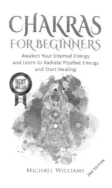

- ***Mindfulness for Beginners*** *- How to Live in The Present, Stress and Anxiety Free*

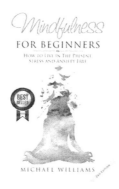

- **Mindfulness:** *An Eight-Step Guide to Finding Peace and Removing Negativity From Your Everyday Life*

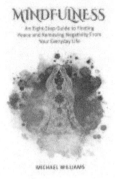

- **Mindfulness For Beginners** - *How to Relieve Stress and Anxiety Like a Buddhist Monk and Live In the Present Moment In Your Everyday Life*

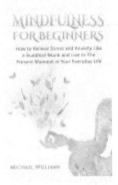

- **Yoga For Men:** *Beginner's Step by Step Guide to a Stronger Body & Sharper Mind*

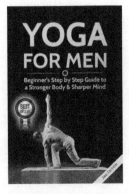

- ***Empath:*** *How to Stop Worrying and Eliminate Negative Thinking as a Sensitive Person*

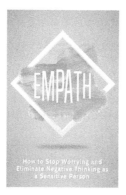

- ***ZEN:*** *Beginner's Guide to Understanding & Practicing Zen Meditation to Become Present*

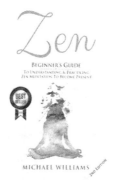

Resources

https://www.care2.com/greenliving/12-yoga-tips-for-beginners.html

http://cloudnineecigreviews.com/health-self-help/yoga-for-male-libido-enhancement-and-sexual-health/

http://www.onepowerfulword.com/2010/10/18-benefits-of-deep-breathing-and-how.html

https://www.artofliving.org/in-en/yoga/yoga-benefits

Made in the USA
Las Vegas, NV
02 October 2024

96119582R00059